ZENECA

First on Call for Urology

Robert K. Carruthers, ChM, FRCS, FRCS(E)
Kent and Canterbury Hospital
Canterbury, Kent CT1 3NG, England

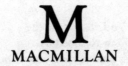

MACMILLAN

First published 1991 by
THE MACMILLAN PRESS LTD
Houndmills, Basingstoke, Hampshire RG21 2XS
and London
Companies and representatives
throughout the world

ISBN 0–333–54820–5

A catalogue record for this book is available
from the British Library.

Printed in Great Britain by
Mackays of Chatham PLC
Chatham, Kent

Reprinted 1994

To J. T., whose life
was ruined by
careless urethral instrumentation

Contents

Preface

This handbook is not intended to be a textbook of urology. Its purpose is to provide young doctors, new to urology, with assistance in dealing with the practical problems, specific to urology, that they may meet during the course of their duties as "first on call" to the Accident and Emergency Department and the ward.

It is fully expected that the protocols and techniques described here will be modified according to local conditions, facilities and preferences. Also, it is assumed that, as the reader becomes more experienced, so individual variations and modifications will be adopted. Until such expertise has been acquired, however, this text will help to answer the question "What do I do next?"

The book is also designed to act as a notebook in which to enter your own observations and schedules, and to record local policies, treatment protocols, etc.

Canterbury, June 1990 R.K.C.

Acknowledgements

I am greatly indebted to my secretary, Mrs Polly Osborne, for her invaluable assistance. The many hours of typing, correcting and retyping the manuscript represent a major contribution, which I acknowledge with gratitude.

Introduction

Urological practice has advanced dramatically during recent years. This is principally due to the progress that has been made in instrument design and in the development of fibre optics and lenses. These advances have, in turn, made access to the renal tract a more sophisticated and precise process, resulting in techniques of surgery that are infinitely less traumatic and distressing to the patient. These advances demanded the development of specialist urological units, and such units now exist in most hospitals throughout the country.

In the past urological emergencies were often regarded as rather an unwelcome part of the general surgical work load; they were reluctantly admitted to general wards and the subsequent treatment was usually fairly major and traumatic. The situation is now different and urological patients are admitted to urological wards and attended to by nurses and doctors trained specifically in urological practices. They benefit from the advances in instrument design and surgical techniques that offer effective surgery for a wider range of conditions and to a much older and less physically fit group of patients. To this extent, urological patients have changed and this change has put greater demands on the doctors and nurses responsible for their hospital treatment. He or she is older, more frail, more knowledgeable and, consequently, more demanding than before and it is therefore even more important that simple routine treatments such as catheterisation, irrigation, etc., be properly understood and properly carried out. A blocked catheter in a fit man aged 60 is painful and distressing but in an 85-year-old with an inadequate myocardium it could be fatal. It is not enough to confidently know that such procedures are necessary; it is essential that you develop a practical expertise in their execution. Confidence without competence is a recipe for disaster.

Urological problems affect patients from all walks of life and from all age groups but there is inevitably a preponderance of the more elderly male patient since a large proportion of urological problems tend to occur at a more advanced age and to concern the male genitourinary tract.

Much of your practical urological work in a busy general hospital will involve the treatment of problems that result from prostatic enlargement, benign or malignant, and the various malignant tumours of the renal tract. You will come to know your patients well, since many of these conditions, though rarely completely curable, are often controllable and therefore demand repeated assessment at intervals, e.g. tumours of the bladder, cancer of the prostate, stone formation, strictures, etc.

The patients, in turn, will come to know and rely on you as their most available and approachable medical ally. They will turn to you as an interpreter of the complexities of medical jargon, techniques and treatment policies. They will depend on you for reassurance, and although your seniors will determine over-all and long-term policy, you are the doctor who solves their immediate problems and anxieties.

Communication with urological patients may occasionally present a challenge, since they are often very old and suffer from a multitude of additional problems, all of which must be assessed and taken into account when prescribing treatment. A precise account of their symptoms is often difficult to elicit. It is a simple enough matter to obtain a history from a young intelligent patient who has all his faculties and who can understand your questions and answer precisely, but unfortunately the urological patient does not always fit this description and a different technique of history taking is often required. Many of your patients may be deaf, partially sighted, confused, disorientated, etc. Often they are uncooperative and angry. Patience and tact will be required to obtain the information that you seek. It is well to remember that failure to communicate is the commonest cause of confusion and strife within a hospital, for both the patients and the staff.

In moments of exasperation it may help to reflect that they are of a generation that has survived many crises and have endured many indignities and infirmities; most have been brought up in circumstances that the present generation would regard as untenable but about which they could do nothing. Many have been poorly recompensed for services given and sacrifices made during the course of their lives. They deserve your best help, understanding and respect. Occasionally you will discover that your patients have been skilled and experienced in fascinating occupations that no longer exist. They have a fund of anecdotes and experiences that are a pleasure to listen to if you can find the time. They are, in addition, of a generation that will be genuinely grateful for your attention and assistance.

Part I

In General

(Equipment and Techniques)

1

Catheters

As a junior doctor in urology, your working life may appear to revolve around catheters. Which catheter to use and when. How to cope when they are not working correctly. When to remove them. When to irrigate and with what. Endless questions arise, most of which will probably be answered in the process of acquiring experience, but these sections are intended to resolve some of the problems before you meet them and so help to avoid the painful process of trial and error.

The essential purpose of all catheters is to drain some part of the urinary tract for short or long periods. Some are used also as splints after operations and as temporary urinary diversion techniques until healing takes place. The techniques of catheterisation and the problems that will be met are discussed in Chapter 2. Probably the most frequent practical manoeuvre you will be asked to perform will be to relieve urinary retention. This can be done by using either a urethral catheter or a suprapubic catheter and you will rapidly become knowledgeable about them. Ureteric catheters, stents, nephrostomy catheters, etc., are also often used and your part in their management will also be discussed briefly.

You will become familiar with specialised catheters in the course of your work but the following notes will introduce you to the more commonly used catheters and give you a very brief indication of their uses.

URETHRAL CATHETERS

The time-honoured method of relieving retention of urine is to pass a urethral catheter. The most commonly used urethral catheter is the Foley catheter (named after Dr Frederic Foley in the mid 1930s). The term 'Foley'' indicates that it has an inflatable balloon as a means of retaining it in position (Figure 1). Foley catheters are manufactured in a variety of materials (see below). The balloon capacity varies and the volume required for inflation is marked on the catheter. You should use the smallest capacity

3

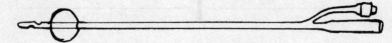

Figure 1   A Foley catheter.

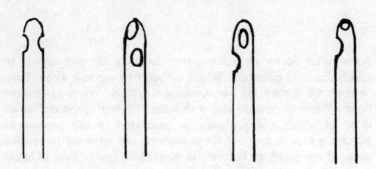

Figure 2   Examples of catheter tips.

balloon (usually 5–10 ml) that will retain the catheter in position—the larger balloons may be necessary under specific circumstances, such as after transurethral surgery. The external diameter of the catheter is indicated by Charriere gauge (marked Ch.) or French gauge (marked Fr). 10 Fr is equivalent to 3.3 mm; 20 Fr is equivalent to 6.6 mm. The eyes or holes at the end or tip of the catheter vary in number, size and position (Figure 2). The shape of the catheter tip may be straight or slightly curved, i.e. Coudé (Figure 3) and Bicoudé (Figure 4). The length of a standard male Foley catheter is approximately 38 cm, but shorter catheters are available, one of approximately 22 cm in length for females and a paediatric catheter of approximately 25 cm.

Latex Foley Catheters

All sizes are available, each with a variety of tip styles, eye portions and balloon sizes. They are fairly soft, relatively cheap and suitable for initial catheterisation in cases of uncomplicated

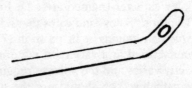

Figure 3   A Coudé catheter tip.

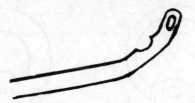

Figure 4   A Bicoudé catheter tip.

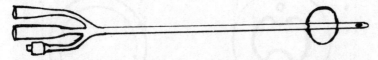

Figure 5   A standard three-way latex Foley catheter.

retention. Use 14 Fr or 16 Fr two-way catheters unless these prove to be too big. They are not advisable for cases which will require bladder syringe suction, because the lumen tends to collapse when negative pressure is applied. They are not suitable for use as long-term indwelling catheters (see p. 21), since they tend to allow encrustation to form on their surfaces and also encourage debris to form in the bladder, which, in turn, causes catheter blockage. Also they are often responsible for stricture formation if left *in situ* for long periods. Two-way catheters and three way catheters are available, but latex catheters are best avoided if irrigation is required, because a standard three-way latex Foley catheter (Figures 5 and 6b) usually has a much smaller outflow channel than a three-way plastic catheter (Figure 6a) of the same external calibre.

It should be mentioned briefly here that some latex catheters are manufactured from high-modulus latex and some which incorporate nylon winding in the wall. These modifications make them stiffer and thus capable of effectively supporting a larger internal lumen. They are also less likely to collapse during suction. A further modification is the latex catheter coated with Teflon. This effectively reduces the likelihood of encrustation and stricture formation.

Plastic Foley Catheters

These are not usually used for initial catheterisation except in a case of clot retention (see p. 69). They are relatively stiff and therefore potentially damaging to the urethra during introduction. They are, however, the best catheters to use if suction is necessary

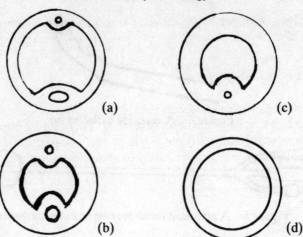

Figure 6   (a) Cross-section of a three-way catheter. (b) Cross-section of a three-way latex Foley catheter, showing the reduced-diameter outflow channel. (c) Cross-section of a silicone two-way Foley catheter. (d) Cross-section of a Jacques or Nélaton single-lumen catheter.

or if irrigation is required, since the outflow lumen of a three-way plastic catheter is relatively larger than that in the equivalent standard latex catheter and they do not tend to collapse when suction is applied. If suction and irrigation are required, use a 20 Fr or 22 Fr catheter.

Silicone Foley Catheters

Two varieties exist (Figure 6c): the pure silicone catheter and the silicone elastomer-coated catheter. The latter is slightly the cheaper of the two, but both are expensive and should not be used for initial short-term catheterisation. These catheters are usually coloured green, blue or white. They are mainly for use as long-term indwelling catheters, and since their surface is made of silicone, they tend not to create debris or block as commonly as a latex catheter. The manufacturers suggest that they can remain *in situ* for approximately 12 weeks. Use a 14 Fr or a 16 Fr catheter for long-term drainage.

Hydrogel Encapsulated Foley Catheters

Relatively new in the UK and rather expensive but very suitable for long-term indwelling catheter drainage. Said to be biocompatible and, hence, to result in less urethritis and stricture formation.

Gibbon Catheters

This is a fine plastic catheter held in the bladder by external flanges which are taped to the penis (Figure 7). There is no Foley balloon. Theoretically they are good but in fact they prove difficult to maintain *in situ*. They are rarely used in everyday practice but are

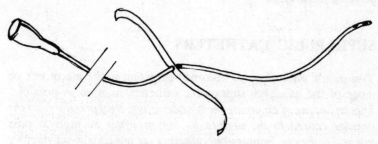

Figure 7   A Gibbons catheter.

worth knowing about. They can sometimes be passed through a strictured urethra when other catheters fail, mainly because they are relatively stiff despite their narrow gauge.

Jacques or Nélaton Catheters

These are narrow straight single-lumen plastic catheters (Figures 6d and 8). They are very suitable for emptying the bladder and then withdrawing straight away—they have no self-retaining device. They may be short or long, for female and male, respectively.

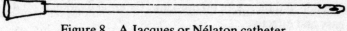

Figure 8   A Jacques or Nélaton catheter.

The short catheter is often used for intermittent self-catheterisation in the female and the long Nélaton catheter may be used as a ureteric splint during and after operation.

Tiemann Catheters

These are manufactured with or without a Foley balloon. They have an olivary tapered end and are rather stiff (Figure 9). They

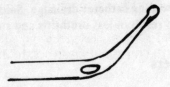

Figure 9   The tip of a Tiemann catheter.

are not recommended for routine use, because of the danger of piercing the urethra.

SUPRAPUBIC CATHETERS

You should endeavour to become competent in the use of one or more of the available suprapubic catheters as soon as possible. *This technique of emptying the bladder is infinitely preferable to the damage caused to the urethra by inappropriate attempts to pass urethral catheters*. Suprapubic catheters are not usually satisfactory for permanent or long-term bladder drainage but are very suitable for short periods.

There are many types of suprapubic catheters currently available. The following are commonly used but the list is not intended to be exhaustive. New designs appear frequently.

Suprapubic Emergency Catheters (S.P.E.C. 5) (Porges)

These catheters are relatively fine and atraumatic (Figure 10). They are inserted by means of a central trocar needle. Since they are of small calibre, they are suitable for short-term use only. They have a Malecot device at the proximal end and are made of polyamide and therefore do not kink. External fixation is relatively easy and effective.

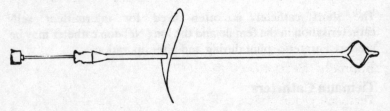

Figure 10   A suprapubic emergency catheter (S.P.E.C.5, Porges).

Silastic Cysto-cath (Dow Corning)

These are made of silicone elastomer and therefore unlikely to kink (Figure 11). They are inserted after a trocar and cannula have

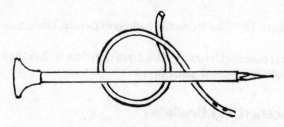

Figure 11   A silastic Cysto-cath (Dow Corning).

first been introduced into the bladder. They are useful if fairly long-term drainage is required. They have good external fixation.

Ingram (Argyle)

These are made of plastic material and are introduced by means of a solid obdurator. They are held in by means of a Foley balloon and a flange stitched to the skin (Figure 12). Various gauges are

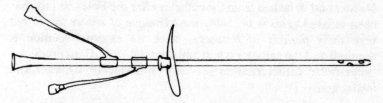

Figure 12   The Ingram catheter (Argyle).

available. They are useful for prolonged drainage but are cumbersome on the surface. Use a very fine needle to inflate the Foley balloon (which regrettably does not have a Luer lock at the inflation end) and so prevent slow leakage from the balloon.

Bonnano (Becton Dickinson)

These are pigtail Teflon catheters inserted by means of a needle obdurator (Figure 13). Very useful for short-term drainage. The pigtail is not sufficiently strong to hold it in the bladder without

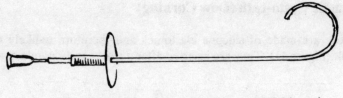

Figure 13   The Bonnano catheter (Becton Dickinson).

additional external fixation. The main criticism is that they tend to kink, block and occasionally break.

Add-a-cath (Cory Brothers)

A relatively recent design (Nottingham introducer) that allows the use of a standard urethral Foley catheter (Figure 14). The catheter

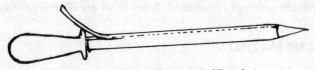

Figure 14   The Add-a-cath (Cory).

is introduced after the insertion of a trocar and sheath. The sheath has a removable strip which enables it to be withdrawn from the bladder and detached from the catheter after the Foley balloon has been inflated. *This is probably the technique of choice for all but very short periods of drainage*, since no external fixation is required and the catheter is soft and does not kink. Bard produce a "suprapubic catheterisation set" with introducers, catheter and instructions.

URETERIC CATHETERS

Ureteric catheters are employed frequently in theatre. You will not be called upon to use them on the ward or in the Accident and Emergency Department. If you are required to use them in theatre, you will be taught the techniques involved. They are used for diagnostic or drainage purposes and are usually placed in position in the course of cystocopy.

Acorn Type—Braasch or Chevassu

These catheters are used in theatre at cystoscopy to obtain an ascending ureteropyelogram (Figure 15). The expanded end is

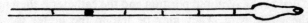

Figure 15 A Braasch or Chevassu acorn-type catheter.

placed in the ureteric orifice and radio-opaque dye is injected into the ureter and hence into the pelvicalyceal system. The X-rays are taken in theatre, often making use of the image intensifier.

Ureteric Whistle Tip Catheters

These catheters are used to introduce radio-opaque dye into the renal pelvis when a pyelogram, but not a ureterogram, is required (Figure 16). The catheter may be passed up the ureter and into the renal pelvis at cystoscopy and the patient may be moved to the

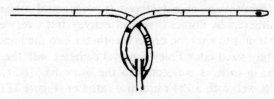

Figure 16 A ureteric whistle-tip catheter.

X-ray department for screening. They may also be used as a temporary indwelling drain to the renal pelvis in cases of ureteric obstruction, or as a splint or stent following ureteric surgery.

Pigtail Stents (J-stents)

Stents are used to drain obstructed kidneys. The coiled "pigtail" serves as a self-retaining device in the renal pelvis (Figure 17). They may be single-ended or double-ended pigtail. The single-

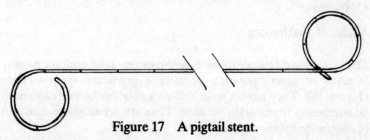

Figure 17 A pigtail stent.

ended pigtail coils in the renal pelvis and the lower end is brought out via the bladder and urethra to the surface. The double-ended pigtail coils both in the renal pelvis and (the lower end) in the bladder and does not drain on to the surface. A guide wire is passed first to the required position and the catheter is then passed over the guide wire. They may be left in the ureter for many weeks.

If the ureteric catheters are to remain *in situ* for a few days, pigtail stents are usually used. However, other catheters may be employed and they are maintained in position by various techniques that will be decided on at the time of operation. If they emerge from the patient via the abdominal wall, they are usually stitched in position. If the catheter passes out via the urethra, it is usual to tape it firmly to an indwelling small calibre urethral Foley catheter.

Occasionally there may be difficulty in maintaining a connection between the narrow ureteric catheter and the wide tube of the urine bag. There are now many specially designed connections available from several manufacturers (the universal connector for ureteric catheters by Porges is very effective), but a very effective D.I.Y. system is to pass the ureteric catheter into the lumen of an appropriately sized latex Foley urethral catheter with the end cut off, which, in turn, is connected to the urine bag (6 Fr ureteric catheter fits well with a 12 Fr urethral catheter (Figure 18)).

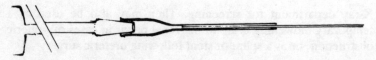

Figure 18   D.I.Y. technique using an appropriately sized latex Foley catheter between the wide tube of a urine bag and a narrow ureteric catheter.

RENAL CATHETERS (Nephrostomy or Pyelostomy Catheters)

Malecot Catheters

These are used frequently as a nephrostomy tube and are usually inserted at open operation or after a percutaneous procedure (Figure 19). They have a weak self-retaining device and require to be stitched in to maintain position. They are occasionally used as a bladder suprapubic catheter.

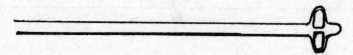

Figure 19   A Malecot catheter.

Cummings Catheter

A Malecot catheter with a narrow ureteric extension (Figure 20), which is used as a nephrostomy tube when splinting of the ureter is also required, e.g. after a difficult pyeloplasty or ureterotomy.

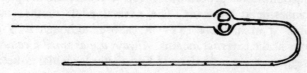

Figure 20   A Cummings Malecot catheter.

2

Catheterisation

URETHRAL CATHETERISATION

The urethra is an extremely sensitive structure and catheterisation is an uncomfortable procedure: therefore you should use plenty of local anaesthetic lubricant. The normal adult urethra usually measures approximately 28 Fr in calibre, although it is often narrower at the external meatus. *Always use as small a catheter as will be effective*, e.g. a 14 Fr or 16 Fr catheter for initial catheterisation. *You must never use force*—if difficulties arise, you must try a smaller-gauge catheter or perform a suprapubic catheterisation. *There is never any justification for being overzealous. It takes only a second to damage a urethra, but to the patient this may mean a lifetime of micturition difficulties, repeated instrumentation and hospitalisation.*

Always explain to the patient what you intend to do and always ensure that you and your equipment are fully organised before you start. This procedure may make or break the patient's confidence.

Catheterisation of the Male Patient

It is essential that the catheter should be passed in a sterile fashion. This does not mean that very prolonged and extensive preparation is required before commencing, but it does mean that any part of the catheter that passes into the urethra must be, and remain, sterile. The following technique is suggested:

1. Wash your hands and open the prepacked catheterisation set. Tear a small hole in paper sheet provided and pass the penis through the hole. Wrap a swab around the penis. Retract the prepuce if necessary and thoroughly clean the glans with cotton wool soaked in Savlon.

2. Squeeze a full tube of lignocaine gel into the urethra, using the nozzle supplied, and occlude the distal urethra by digital pressure or apply a penile clamp (Figure 21) to retain the lignocaine in the urethra—where it is needed. Take the catheter from its outer covering.

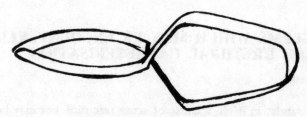

Figure 21 A penile clamp, used to retain lignocaine in the urethra.

3. Remove the penile clamp and put on sterile gloves. Hold the penis up and pass the catheter carefully and slowly. You should avoid contact with the catheter itself: touch only the inner sleeve cover of the catheter—sometimes it is useful to apply a spinning action to the catheter as it advances up the urethra. The inner sleeve cover is removed concertina fashion as the catheter is passed. A "no touch technique" is desirable even though you are wearing sterile gloves.
4. Inflate the Foley balloon to the required volume, using sterile water only (balloon size marked on catheter). Ensure that the prepuce, if present, is forward and so avoid a paraphimosis. Take a specimen of urine for bacterial culture and for routine ward testing. *Always record the volume of urine obtained and note if it is blood stained. Make a note of any difficulty experienced.*

Catheterisation of the Female Patient

This, in practice, is often performed by the nursing staff but achieving a sterile catheterisation may be more difficult than it is in the male. The labia must be held apart and careful swabbing of the labia majora and minora must be carried out, using an anterior to posterior movement and discarding the swab after each movement. Finally, swab the central region of the vulva and the urethral meatus. If the catheter is to be left *in situ* for only a short time, the standard latex Foley catheter will suffice, but if a longer term is envisaged you should remember that shorter (female) Foley catheters are available and may be more comfortable.

PROBLEMS WHICH MAY BE ENCOUNTERED DURING URETHRAL CATHETERISATION
Phimosis

This is rarely, in itself, a cause of acute retention but may be an associated condition. The tight prepuce may make it difficult or impossible for you to find the external urethral meatus and so will prevent catheterisation. Occasionally you may be able to stretch the phimosis sufficiently with an artery forcep to expose the meatus, but this exercise will probably be too painful.

A "dorsal slit" of the prepuce is necessary in most cases. For this a local anaesthetic subcutaneous ring block is used (lignocaine 1% or Marcain 0.5% without adrenaline (Figure 22)). With scissors or

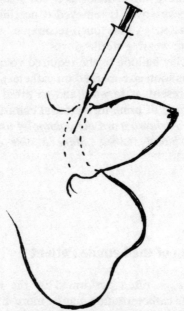

Figure 22   Diagram to show position and application of a
subcutaneous ring block.

a scalpel blade, the prepuce overlying the dorsum of the glans is then cut just sufficiently to allow exposure of the meatus (Figure 23).

If the phimosis cannot be dealt with adequately in this way, you should use a suprapubic catheter (see p. 19).

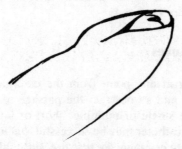

Figure 23   Diagram to show incision of the dorsum of the glans to expose the meatus.

Paraphimosis

This occurs when a relatively tight prepuce has been pulled back proximal to the glans and has not been returned to its normal position. The prepuce in the new position forms a tight band around the corona, resulting in local oedema. The glans and foreskin distal to the constricting band become congested and swollen. The longer treatment is delayed, the more difficult it is to effect an easy cure.

Occasionally the paraphimosis may be reduced (a) manually by manipulating the constricting band forward after gentle and prolonged squeezing of the glans to reduce the congestion. If this technique fails it will be necessary (b) to accurately cut through the constricting band at the dorsal aspect of the penis immediately proximal to the glans with a scalpel blade, using a local anaesthetic

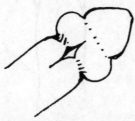

Figure 24   Diagram to show incision of the constricting band to reduce paraphimosis (dorsal slit).

subcutaneous ring block (Figure 24). (c) Formal circumcision will be required at a later stage even if the paraphimosis has been successfully reduced. If facilities exist for circumcision straight away, then this is probably the best course, since it treats both the paraphimosis and the underlying phimosis. Circumcision can equally well be done under general or local anaesthetic. Full theatre facilities are required.

Urethral Strictures

These may occur at any point from the external meatus to the prostatic urethra and so obstruct the passage of a catheter. The strictures may be single or multiple, short or long. Occasionally the use of a finer catheter may be successful, *but no attempt should be made to forcibly negotiate the stricture*, since false passages may be created which considerably worsen the condition. Do not attempt to dilate the strictures by the use of sounds or bougies, as this is a task for more experienced members of the urology staff. *Suprapubic catheterisation is, without doubt, the manoeuvre of choice.*

Hypospadias

Beware of the unsuspected hypospadias in the adult. Do not try to catheterise the "false dimple" that may masquerade as the external urinary meatus. The real meatus may be centimetres away on the ventral aspect of the penis (Figure 25). The patient may not be aware of any abnormality!

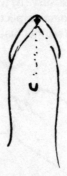

Figure 25   A false dimple may be some distance from the real meatus.

SUPRAPUBIC CATHETERISATION

You must adopt this method of draining the bladder without hesitation if urethral catheterisation proves difficult for any reason, but beware the patient who has had lower abdominal or pelvic surgery in the past.

One of the inadequacies of the suprapubic catheter is its tendency to kink and break on the surface of the abdomen. Also, they are liable to be pulled out accidentally by patient or nurse. Usually such accidents can be prevented by careful attention to the technique of fixing the catheter on to the abdominal skin. Time spent on this task is seldom wasted and ingenuity should be used to fix the catheter and its drainage tube firmly.

Technique

Sterile technique is essential. Suprapubic catheters are prepacked and each pack contains specific instructions on their individual use. It is essential that you read these instructions and follow them carefully. If the techniques described are correctly executed, there should be no difficulty. However, the following additional tips are well worth emphasising:

1. In most cases where a suprapubic catheter is required, the distended bladder will be easily palpable and usually visible. Nevertheless, it is vital to verify that what you can see and feel is, in fact, the bladder and that it contains urine. This may be achieved by the following simple and safe procedure.

    (i) Clean the suprapubic skin, and select a point approximately 5 cm above the pubic symphysis and in the mid-line.
    (ii) Using lignocaine 1% in a 10 ml syringe and a 21 gauge 1½ in "green" needle, slowly insert the needle at right angles to the skin, anaesthetising the tissues in the process.
    (iii) When the needle is completely buried and all the local anaesthetic has been expelled, withdraw the plunger of the syringe: you should obtain urine.
    (iv) If you do, make a small incision in the skin and rectus sheath with a No. 11 or No. 15 knife blade and proceed with the technique of introducing the catheter according to the instructions contained in the pack.
    (v) If urine is not obtained, *do not proceed—ask for help*.

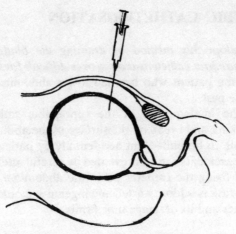

Figure 26   Technique employed to confirm the presence of a full
bladder.

2. The S.P.E.C. 5, the Ingram and the Bonnano catheters are
   introduced with a central pointed obdurator. It is an important
   point of technique not to withdraw the obdurator from the
   catheter until the catheter has been "railroaded" down the
   obdurator well into the bladder. If the obdurator has been
   removed too soon, the catheter cannot easily be advanced
   further into the bladder and it is often impossible to reintroduce
   the obdurator needle into the catheter without damaging it.

CATHETER INTRODUCERS

Catheter introducers are used when it is necessary to have greater
directional control over the catheter as it traverses the urethra.
*They are not intended to be a means of forcing a catheter through a
stricture or other obstruction.*

   They are of particular assistance when passing a plastic catheter
after the completion of a prostatectomy, since the relatively rigid
nature of the catheter may otherwise cause it to pass under the
bladder neck or trigone. The catheter may even pierce the
prostatic capsule if it is not directed correctly and gently into the
bladder.

   *Introducers should only be used after suitable demonstration and
under careful supervision. They are very dangerous if the user is
inexperienced.*

Maryfield Introducer

This is a rigid curved metal strip which is also curved or grooved in cross-section (Figure 27). The tip of the introducer is placed in the

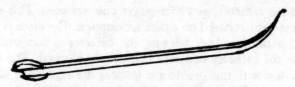

Figure 27 A Maryfield introducer.

eye of the catheter, which is then stretched along the grooved convex surface of the introducer. Once the catheter has been passed into the bladder, the introducer is removed by slipping the tip out of the eye of the catheter. Adequate lubrication is vital, both within the urethra and between the catheter and the introducer. There are three sizes.

Wire Introducer (Clutton Curve)

This is a moderately stiff wire which is inserted into the lumen of the catheter (Figure 28). It is less rigid than a Maryfield introducer and is therefore less dangerous, but it provides much less directional control.

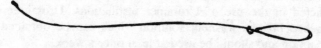

Figure 28 A wire introducer (Clutton curve).

LONG-TERM INDWELLING CATHETERS

Long-term indwelling catheters present many problems and are therefore *only acceptable if there is no alternative*. They are valuable in patients (a) who develop retention but are considered unfit for surgery, (b) who decline the offer of surgery or (c) whose retention persists despite surgery. They are also used commonly in patients who are hopelessly incontinent, although in these patients it is much better if an external incontinence sheath can be used; these appliances, unfortunately, are not always suitable or effective, and therefore an indwelling catheter is often the only practical alternative.

A 16–18 Fr silicone Foley catheter should be used. There is no advantage in using larger-gauge catheters. Occasionally you may be told that the catheter was "leaking", i.e. urine was passing around the catheter, and so a bigger one was used. This wish to "plug the gap" is based on a false assumption. The urine is passed around a catheter, not because the catheter is too small, but because the catheter becomes temporarily blocked. The correct way to deal with this problem is to clear the bladder of accumulated debris. This may sometimes be accomplished by simply washing the bladder out, using saline and a bladder syringe. However, if blockage occurs frequently, it may be necessary to use a cystoscope or resectoscope and an Ellik's evacuator. This is best done as an arranged procedure in the operating theatre with a local or general anaesthetic. Cystoscopy should be performed at the same time, to ensure that all the offending debris has been removed.

The catheter is normally connected to a urine bag to achieve constant drainage and so to ensure an empty bladder. Alternatively, a spigot or a tap can be fitted and the patient can be instructed to drain the bladder when necessary and convenient. The Staubli valve (Figure 29) has recently been introduced and has been constructed in such a way that it may be used by patients with very limited manual dexterity. If used correctly, it allows the normal filling cycle of the bladder to occur and this, theoretically, prevents bladder shrinkage.

Patients must be encouraged to take a large fluid intake and be instructed in the use of Urotainer instillations. Urotainer is a prepacked bladder-washout solution which can be obtained on prescription and should be used at least once a week.

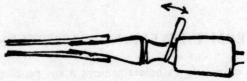

Figure 29   A Staubli valve.

3

Urine Bags

The following types of urine bag are available:

Leg bag The bag (Figure 30) is strapped to the leg in whatever position is most comfortable for the patient. Suitable for a chair-bound patient but rather cumbersome for the ambulant, although some patients find it satisfactory.

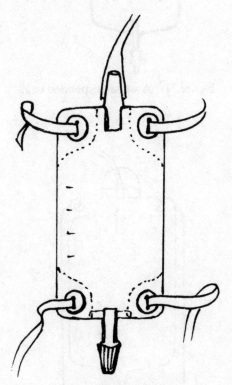

Figure 30   A leg bag.

Waist-suspended bag The bag (Figure 31) is suspended from a belt around the patient's waist (Porta system). This is much the best system for the mobile patient.

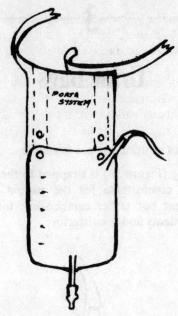

Figure 31   A waist-suspended bag.

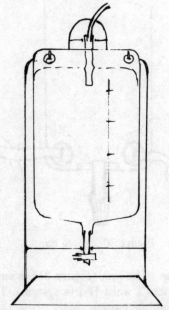

Figure 32   An overnight urine bag.

Overnight urine bag, e.g. the S4 Uribag These are best for the bed-bound patient (Figure 32). They have a large capacity (2–4 litres) and a special S4 bag stand is available.

All of these bags have taps which allow them to be emptied when full without disconnecting the bag from the catheter. There are, of course, as many varieties of these urine bags as there are manufacturers.

4

Bladder Irrigation

Bladder irrigation is commonly used (though not essential) after any operation that causes blood to accumulate within the bladder or the prostatic cavity. It is useful following both transurethral and open surgery. The object of the irrigation is to remove blood from the bladder *before* it can accumulate and clot. Thus, it should be used to prevent clotting and not be regarded as a means of washing clots out after they have formed.

Irrigating fluid should be isotonic. Glycine 1.5% is normally used during transurethral operations, being non-conductive, and normal saline is used during the post-operative period. Isotonic solutions are desirable, since there is almost inevitably a variable volume of irrigating fluid absorbed during the course of an operation through the venous plexuses which lie in and around the prostatic capsule. If water or hypotonic fluid were to be used and absorbed, intravascular lysis of blood cells could occur.

Irrigation of the bladder is usually performed through a three-way latex urethral catheter (Figure 5) which allows an inflow and an outflow at the same time, through the same catheter. Alternatively, a suprapubic catheter may be used as an inflow route for the irrigation fluid and a two-way urethral catheter may be used for outflow. This has the advantage that a two-way catheter has a wider outflow lumen than a three-way catheter of similar external gauge (Figure 6).

It is important that the process of irrigation be carefully monitored by the nursing staff. This presents problems in under-staffed wards. Irrigation, to be effective, must be continuous, and therefore large volumes are involved, which, in turn, means that the urine bags must be emptied frequently. The irrigation fluid should be warmed to approximately body temperature; otherwise, the patient will rapidly lose heat as litre after litre of cold fluid is passed through the bladder.

The rate of irrigation is adjusted so that blood is effectively washed out. Beware of the irrigation that suddenly becomes quite clear after a haemorrhagic operation. This usually suggests that the irrigation fluid is not circulating sufficiently within the bladder to pick up and wash out the blood. Readjusting the position of the catheter within the bladder usually corrects the fault.

5

Urethral Dilators

In most cases urethral strictures will be dealt with in the operating theatre or day unit by means of urethroscopy and direct vision urethrotomy. However, there are occasions when simple urethral dilation is appropriate, since this can be done immediately and using local anaesthetic. *It is a technique that you should use only after demonstration and repeated supervision, since it is possible to cause great harm if done incorrectly. It is essential that dilatation be performed gently and with great care—force should never be used.*

There are three commonly used urethral dilators:

1. Curved metal sounds—e.g. Clutton (Figure 33) or Lister's (Figure 34). These are used to dilate strictures located in the proximal and membraneous urethra.

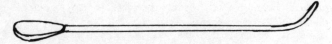

Figure 33   A Clutton urethral dilator.

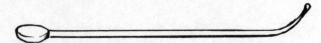

Figure 34   A Lister's urethral dilator.

2. Straight gum-elastic bougies, used to dilate strictures in the anterior urethra (Figure 35).
3. "Follow-on" gum-elastic bougies (Figure 36). These are extremely useful when a stricture is tight or when there are already established false passages. Several of the extremely fine

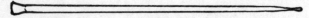

Figure 35   A straight gum-elastic bougie.

28

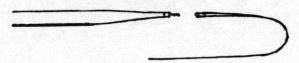

Figure 36   A "follow-on" gum-elastic bougie.

(filiform) "leader" bougies are passed until one of them finds the correct hole in the stricture and passes onward into the bladder. The "followers" are then screwed on to the filiform leader and the combined bougie is pushed gently through the stricture and into the bladder.

Use sterile technique as previously outlined for the passage of a urethral catheter (see p. 14).

Plenty of anaesthetic gel should be employed and, using a penile clamp, allow time for it to take effect before starting to dilate (see Figure 21).

Antibiotic cover may be desirable if the patient has a history of rigors, etc., following previous dilatation.

Finally, and again, *never use force but seek assistance if the dilatation proves to be difficult. Do not use urethral dilators to enable you to pass a urethral catheter, but always employ a suprapubic catheter and leave the urethra strictly alone if the catheter will not pass easily.*

Part II

In the Ward

(Management of Acute Post-operative and Other Problems)

6

Introduction to the Urology Ward

Work in the urology ward requires a variety of talents—talents that can cope with a wide spectrum of problems, from the management of a dramatic post-operative haemorrhage to the more tactful explanations needed to give confidence to an apprehensive patient.

Try to remember your patients by name. Talk to them about their forthcoming operation. They do not know what to expect during the post-operative period following, for example, their prostate operation. Explain that blood transfusion may be necessary, and a catheter will be present and that irrigation may be used. They are not aware that it is common to develop slight haematuria a week or so after they go home and that this is not a cause for alarm but will probably cease after a day or so. If they are to have an orchidectomy, explain the reasons for it and its effect. If they have been admitted with colic, explain the expected series of events as the suspected stone passes down the ureter and the possible alternatives to a "wait and see" policy. Conversations of this nature help to promote confidence and equanimity. Also, listen carefully to their complaints. This might save lengthy investigations, e.g. urodynamics, which can be invasive, embarrassing and inconclusive.

Try to be available to relatives. This contact is always desirable, and a great deal of anxiety can be removed by a few words to wives, sons or daughters. In some cases this communication is more than just desirable: it is essential.

Be aware that variation in the attitude of patients towards their medical problems is enormous. Some wish to have detailed explanations; others prefer to be left in ignorance. This is especially so with regard to the diagnosis of cancer. You will be doing the patient no service in forcing unwelcome information on him if his personality is such that it will cause great depression and withdrawal. On the other hand, it is often necessary to give quite detailed information if the patient is to understand the need for further therapy, e.g. chemotherapy or radiotherapy. Similarly, it is clearly quite wrong to withhold details of diagnosis and prognosis from a patient who genuinely wishes to know. Learn to assess a patient's attitude, anxieties, character, etc., as quickly as possible, so that you may be able to manage these difficult problems with kindness and maturity. Whatever is told or not told to the patient, it is important that someone in the immediate family be acquainted with the facts.

You must learn quickly to assimilate the details of your patient's medical history—many urological conditions are treated by a variety of methods, e.g. surgery, radiotherapy, intravesical instillation, chemotherapy, etc., and it is essential to know which methods have been used in the past so that current and future treatment can be planned.

Always remember that laboratory tests and X-rays are costly and time-consuming. Ask only for those that are necessary and be sure that, if you have requested a test, you see the result and communicate it to others if necessary.

Write legible notes—they should be relevant and without padding. Write drug charts clearly and think ahead, e.g. about night sedation. Effective sleep is essential for recovery. This may not be easy to achieve. Sleeplessness may occur for a variety of reasons, e.g. pain, anxiety, noise, disturbance of sleep rhythm, lack of daytime exercise, etc. The cause should be sought and effective treatment should be given. Patients always feel better after a good sleep.

Learn to manage post-operative drains. Usually drains are only of value if they are draining. When the drainage has been reduced to a minimum, they should, as a rule, be removed. However, it is best to check with your seniors.

Throughout your work on the ward you should also be learning, but do not expect to be "spoon-fed". Question and answer is a very important technique of learning, but reading is also essential. Standard texts should be studied so that questions may be asked within the background of a sound basic knowledge. The benefit derived from your questions will then be much greater.

Remember also that you are not expected to know everything so do not try to manage cases beyond your capabilities. Confer with those more experienced than yourself.

7

The Blocked Catheter

Urethral catheters, unfortunately, do frequently become blocked. The problem occurs commonly in two different circumstances: (1) the long-term indwelling catheter that becomes blocked by accumulated debris (this has already been dealt with on p. 21), or (2) the early post-operative catheter that becomes blocked by blood clot or by loose prostatic or bladder tissue. This does not necessarily mean that there is excessive bleeding, but since it creates many problems for the patient, not the least of which is pain, it should be remedied as soon as possible. If irrigation is being used at the time of blockage, the bladder rapidly fills up and the discomfort becomes intense. The following steps may be helpful in overcoming the problem:

1. Check that the catheter is indeed blocked. Confirm by suprapubic palpation and by briefly disconnecting the urine bag tube from the catheter and allowing the tube to empty. Observe whether the tube refills from the bladder.
2. Check the site of blockage—usually, of course, this is at the eye of the catheter within the bladder, but occasionally blockage owing to clot can occur at the junction of the urine bag and its tube, especially if a bag fitted with a flutter valve is being used.
3. Check that the irrigation fluid is flowing well, or, if it has been intentionally discontinued, that it can flow when required. Occasionally the "stylet" is not pushed adequately into the irrigation fluid bag. Occasionally the clips (taps) are inadvertently shut, or the inflow channel of the three way catheter is inadequate or blocked.
4. If the blockage seems to be in the catheter, check that the catheter is correctly placed in the bladder. The balloon should lie *in* the bladder and not in the prostatic cavity (Figure 37). If there appears to be an inordinate length of catheter outside the urethra, push it gently into the bladder. This manoeuvre may require a little lubrication of the catheter at the meatus and may produce discomfort for the patient. If this move presents any difficulty, deflate the catheter balloon and try again. Usually

35

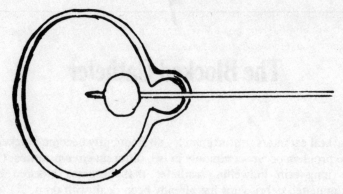

Figure 37   Position the balloon in the bladder, not in the prostatic cavity.

this will have the required effect and the catheter will again drain. Try to wash out any clots that have accumulated and don't forget to reinflate the balloon when the catheter has been properly positioned.

5. If it appears that the catheter is correctly placed within the bladder, it should be possible to clear any accumulated clot from the catheter and from the bladder by aspiration, using a 60 ml bladder syringe. Clot is relatively soft during the early post-operative period and it is usually readily removed by this means.

6. If the use of the syringe is unsuccessful despite ensuring that the catheter is correctly placed, the possibility is that the catheter is blocked by a segment of loose prostatic tissue, and it may be possible to dislodge it by pushing 30–40 ml of saline into the catheter rather than withdrawing it.

7. If this manoeuvre fails, the catheter will probably have to be changed. Catheter changing should not be undertaken lightly. In the post-operative period this procedure may not be simple and it is best to seek more experienced help.

8. If such help is not available it is advisable to use a Coudé catheter or a catheter introducer *but use the latter only if you have had adequate instruction on its use.*

9. Once the catheter has been cleared and the bladder distension relieved, it is important to maintain rapid irrigation and to ensure that the correct catheter position is maintained. This is achieved by an Elastoplast retaining patch on the thigh placed in such a position that only approximately 4 in of catheter is visible outside the urethral meatus.

Isotonic solution, e.g. glycine 1.5% or normal saline, should be used for bladder washout and irrigation. Antibiotics are advisable if there is extensive catheter manipulation.

8

Post-operative Bleeding

If you are called by the nursing staff to the ward or recovery room because of persistent heavy bleeding after a bladder or prostatic operation, you must, straight away, initiate the following procedure:

1. Check the patient's blood pressure and ascertain that there is sufficient blood or plasma expander available for transfusion.
2. Make sure that the bladder is draining well and that it is not distended with either clot or irrigation fluid.
3. Aim to irrigate at a rate sufficient to prevent clotting, but if clots form, they must be syringed out before blockage of the catheter can occur.
4. Check that the catheter is in the correct position, i.e. the balloon must be in the bladder and not in the prostatic cavity (Figure 37). In most cases bleeding will eventually stop provided that the bladder is not distended and provided that it is adequately irrigated.
5. If the bleeding persists despite adequate irrigation, you must check that there is no evidence of a clotting disorder and be

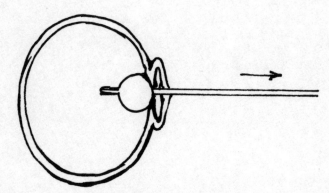

Figure 38   Traction on the catheter may control early post-prostatectomy bleeding.

aware of the possibility of disseminated intravascular coagulation (DIC).

6. Early post-prostatectomy bleeding may sometimes be controlled by traction on the catheter (Figure 38). You must ensure that the catheter balloon contains approximately 40 ml of water and that the balloon is positioned in the bladder and not in the prostatic cavity. A bandage is applied to the leg just below the knee joint, and the catheter is drawn down to this bandage and fixed there by means of a strong elastic band and a safety pin. This has the effect of pulling the catheter balloon down on to the bladder neck and so compressing the prostatic capsule from above, thus, it is to be hoped, occluding the bleeding vessels. Alternatively, the traction may be applied by an orthopaedic weight (0.5 kg) over a pulley at the end of the bed. The traction can be released after 30 min and reapplied if the haemorrhage becomes profuse again. Catheter traction is uncomfortable and the patient should be well sedated.

7. If catheter traction is ineffective, the next step is to return the patient to theatre and search for bleeding points. This decision will be taken after discussion with the surgeon who performed the original operation.

9

DVT and Pulmonary Embolus

DEEP VEIN THROMBOSIS

Most urological patients are, theoretically, in the "high risk" group for post-operative venous thrombosis, i.e. they are old, they often have cardiovascular disorders, they are usually frail and relatively immobile, and they are undergoing pelvic operations. Despite this, it is a post-operative complication that presents surprisingly uncommonly in urological wards.

While it is true to say that there are many cases of DVT and pulmonary emboli which produce no symptoms and therefore go undetected, it is also true that a certain proportion of patients who appear to have the clinical signs of calf vein thrombosis are found, when further investigated, to have normal patent vessels.

The treatment of venous thrombosis or pulmonary embolus is time-consuming and not without its dangers; therefore it is essential that you make a precise diagnosis.

Your main concern is to (a) encourage a scheme of prevention, (b) correctly investigate suspected cases and (c) treat the established condition.

Prevention

If there is a previous history of venous thrombosis, the patient should be given 5000 units heparin (Minihep) subcutaneously, twice daily, starting the night before the operation and continuing 12-hourly thereafter for 5 days. Intermittent calf compression (venous flow stimulators) should be used during surgery, unless the patient is to be in the lithotomy position, and during the post-operative period the patient should wear elasticated stockings (T.E.D.) and ankle movements should be encouraged.

Physiotherapy and early mobilisation should be the aim.

Diagnosis

The diagnosis of deep vein thrombosis is often difficult. A calf vein occlusion may exist on its own or may be associated with more extensive thigh and pelvic vein involvement. Pelvic vein thrombosis may occur with normal patent leg veins.

A calf vein thrombosis may be suspected clinically when there is unilateral swelling of the ankle and foot associated with calf tenderness, a positive Homan's sign and possibly a pyrexia. Typically, a thrombosis of the pelvic vein is relatively symptomless, but it may present with a swollen thigh and calf which the patient feels to be tight and heavy. If the signs and symptoms suggest a DVT and further proof is required, the most valuable diagnostic test is *phlebography*. You should arrange this with the X-ray Department as soon as possible. Interpretation of the radiographs is difficult and discussion with the radiologist is essential. Doppler ultrasound is still sometimes used and has the advantage of being non-invasive, but realise that it is unreliable and may give false negative results. It is only of value if there is massive occlusion of thigh or pelvic veins. Thrombosis in calf vein is not reliably detected.

Treatment of an Established Deep Vein Thrombosis

Elasticated stockings are worn. The bed should be slightly elevated. Knee and ankle movements should be encouraged. Analgesics may be required.

You should commence anticoagulation. The protocol for anticoagulation varies from hospital to hospital but the following regimen is adequate. A loading dose of 5000 units heparin is given intravenously. Thereafter 1000–1500 units heparin are given intravenously per hour by continuous infusion pump for 5 days. It is wise to monitor heparin therapy daily by measuring the A.P.T.T. (activated partial thromboplastin time).

At the same time as the heparin therapy is started, oral warfarin is prescribed. A dose of 10 mg daily is sufficient. PT (prothrombin time) estimations are arranged with the haematologist, who will usually dictate warfarin dosage thereafter and decide the frequency of prothrombin tests. Your aim is to obtain a BCR (British Corrected Ratio) of between 2 and 4.

The half-life of heparin is very short (approximately 2 h), so reversal is seldom required. However, should rapid reversal be necessary, protamine sulphate 25 mg can be used. The dose should not exceed 50 mg.

If it is necessary to reverse warfarin therapy, this is best achieved by intravenous vitamin K (2 mg) and, if necessary, by transfusion of fresh frozen plasma.

Remember that warfarin therapy in the presence of other drugs may be difficult. Many interactions occur and the anticoagulant effect of warfarin may be exaggerated by some and inhibited by other drugs. Question your patients carefully to discover what drugs they are currently taking and then discuss the problem with the haematologist. Drugs of many types may have a significant effect, e.g. analgesics, antibiotics, sedatives, etc.

PULMONARY EMBOLUS

Clinical signs suggestive of pulmonary embolus usually only appear if the vascular obstruction has been fairly extensive. The classical features are haemoptysis, pleuritic pain, breathlessness, cyanosis and raised JVP. ECG changes may occur but are usually non-specific and unreliable. Chest X-ray may help, if only to exclude other pulmonary pathology. The most reliable diagnostic test is an *isotope (technetium) perfusion lung scan* (VQ scan).

Treatment

Anticoagulation therapy as described for deep vein thrombosis is commenced. Oxygen therapy may be necessary, and possibly analgesics. Subsequently streptokinase treatment may be considered. Embolectomy is rarely indicated.

ELECTIVE SURGERY ON ANTICOAGULATED PATIENTS

In view of the age of many of your patients admitted for transurethral surgery, it will not be a surprise to find that some of them have been placed on long-term anticoagulant therapy for previous vascular problems. Warfarin therapy should be discontinued and subcutaneous heparin substituted. The following is a suggested programme for these patients:

1. You should arrange that the patient discontinues warfarin therapy at least 24 h before the proposed operation.
2. The prothrombin time should be estimated as close to the

commencement of the proposed operation as possible and the result should be communicated to both surgeon and anaesthetist before the patient is taken to theatre.

3. Intravenous vitamin K may be used if active rapid reversal of warfarin is required. Fresh frozen plasma should be available if required.

4. 5000 units heparin are given subcutaneously the night before the operation and continued b.d. until the warfarin, which is restarted the morning following the operation (provided that there is no excessive bleeding), has reached therapeutic levels again, as judged by the prothrombin time results.

Prothrombin time estimation is performed by the Pathology Laboratory and warfarin dosage is dictated in the usual way.

10

Slight but Persistent Haematuria

It is assumed that the patient has been cystoscoped and that the cause of the persistent haematuria is known. The problem may arise with, for example, post-radiotherapy telangiectasia, carcinoma of prostate or low-grade widespread bladder tumours. It is assumed also that further cystoscopy is not in the interest of the patient and that conservative means should be employed.

1. You must ensure that the urine is not infected.
2. Check clotting indices such as PT, APTT, platelet count, etc.
3. If clotting factors are abnormal, intravenous vitamin K, an infusion of platelets or fresh frozen plasma may be of value.
4. Catheterisation and irrigation should be used only if clotting is a problem, but be aware that the very presence of the catheter may in some cases be the cause of persistent slight haematuria.
5. Try Cyklokapron (tranexamic acid) 1.5 g t.d.s. orally. This is an antifibrinolytic agent which can also be given intravenously. Cyklokapron should be used for a maximum of 5 days only.
6. If Cyklokapron fails, try Dicynene IG 6-hourly orally. Dicynene acts by maintaining small-vessel integrity but has no direct action on the clotting mechanism. Dicynene should be used for 1 week only.

11

TUR Syndrome

Uncommonly, after transurethral surgery the patient may become confused, uncooperative and hypotensive, and develop a brachy-cardia, sickness and sometimes collapse. This syndrome may be associated with hyponatraemia and hypervolaemia (and possibly hyperammonaemia) and is thought to be due to the absorption of isotonic irrigating fluid during the course of operation and in the post-operative period. The hyperammonaemia results from the metabolic breakdown of absorbed glycine and may be partly responsible for signs of encephalopathy.

The syndrome is rapidly corrected when the irrigation is discontinued, diuretics are prescribed and the sodium deficit is corrected by an infusion of N or 2 N saline (although the latter is rarely needed).

12

Failure of Catheter Balloon to Deflate

Occasionally you may faced with the problem of a Foley catheter that cannot be removed. The cause of this is almost invariably a failure of the Foley balloon to deflate, despite attempts to withdraw the water from the balloon. One of the following procedures may be effective:

1. Occasionally the balloon can be induced to soften and disintegrate if 5 ml of liquid paraffin is introduced into it via the usual inflating channel.
2. If you can obtain a little ether (3 ml), inject it into the balloon of the catheter along the normal inflating channel. The balloon will rapidly disintegrate, spilling the ether (already diluted by the water in the balloon) into the bladder. It is important

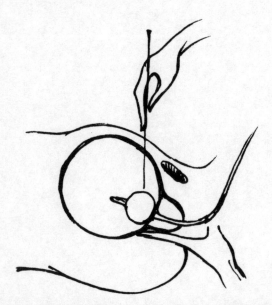

Figure 39   If all else fails, burst the balloon with a lumbar puncture needle.

because of this spillage that the bladder be filled with at least 300 ml of water before introducing the ether and that this be rapidly and completely drained before the catheter is withdrawn.

3. It may be possible to pass the stylet wire of a ureteric catheter along the inflating channel of the catheter until it reaches the balloon. A sharp forward movement then pierces the balloon.

4. If the above techniques fail, the problem will be overcome by locating the balloon within the bladder by rectal palpation with the index finger of one hand, and introducing into the bladder a long thin needle (lumbar puncture needle) under local anaesthetic suprapubically and guiding it with the other hand on to the balloon, thus bursting it and allowing the catheter to be withdrawn (Figure 39).

13

"Catheter Spasm"

A small percentage of patients who have a urethral catheter *in situ* may complain of recurrent episodes of severe pain that is felt in the region of the bladder and urethra. At the same time they may pass urine around the outside of the catheter. The pain is usually short-lived but is very unpleasant and, unfortunately, is very difficult to control. This "spasm" may be relieved by reducing the volume of water in the Foley balloon or on some occasions by employing a smaller calibre of catheter. The most effective treatment is to remove the catheter, but until this is possible, try Pro-Banthine, Buscopan or Urispas. Occasionally Pyridium may be of value.

14

Analgesics

Post-operative pain relief is, on the whole, poorly managed but it is an aspect of care that is essential for the well-being and recovery of the patient. Not all analgesics suit all patients. You should know a variety and have in your mind (or in your notebook) a list of drugs of varying efficacy, for children as well as adults—i.e. drugs varying from the most potent, e.g. morphine, to the less effective, such as co-proxamol, Panadol, etc. Analgesia should be prescribed in adequate doses: there is little value in administering pethidine 50 mg to a 17 stone man with severe renal colic! Don't forget the value of the continuous infusion of drugs such as fentanyl or morphine, although this technique should be confined to high-dependency wards. Patient-controlled anaesthesia (PCA) is a very efficient method of pain control but requires patient selection and careful explanation. Epidural anaesthesia (Marcain), which may be "topped up" at intervals by the indwelling cannula, is also very effective. If in doubt, discuss the problem with the anaesthetists. They have considerable expertise and will be pleased to help.

The following list of analgesics is not exhaustive but the drugs are readily available and are in fairly common use. There are many others.

Low potency

Aspirin
Paracetamol
Indomethacin
Voltarol
Naprosyn

Medium potency

Codeine
Dihydrocodeine

Fortral (pentazocine)
Co-proxamol

High potency

Short duration: pethidine
Medium duration: morphine
                           diamorphine
Long duration: Temgesic (sublingual)

15

Urinary Tract Infection

Most urinary tract infections are caused by organisms that are normal inhabitants of the gut. Often the infections are asymptomatic but occasionally they produce dramatic symptoms in either the upper or the lower urinary tract. The infection is easily diagnosed by routine culture techniques after the collection of a mid-stream or catheter specimen of urine. In a large proportion of cases the infecting organism is a Gram-negative bacillus or enterococcus, e.g. *E. coli*, *Proteus*, *Bacteroides*, *Klebsiella*, *Pseudomonas*, etc., although in hospital practice other organisms occur with increased frequency, e.g. streptococci and staphylococci.

Theoretically, drug treatment should be withheld until an organism has been isolated and identified and sensitivities have been reported. In practice it is reasonable, in most uncomplicated urinary infections, to prescribe a simple antimicrobial agent such as trimethoprim (200 mg b.d.), nitrofurantoin (100 mg t.d.s.) or a sulphonamide (e.g. sulphadimidine 0.5 g t.d.s.) and to modify this therapy when the urine sample has been examined and reported— usually the therapy will not need to be changed.

Occasionally the clinical situation is much more serious and "best guess" antibiotics are urgently required, e.g. in septicaemia. In these cases it is, again, reasonable to assume that the infecting organism is likely to be a Gram-negative bacillus or possibly *Streptococcus faecalis* and to prescribe large doses of parenteral antibiotics immediately, such as gentamicin (120 mg) or a cephalosporin such as cefuroxime (1.5 g), perhaps with ampicillin (500 mg) or erythromycin in the presence of penicillin hypersensitivity. In the case of life-threatening infection, you must be sure to use adequate doses, but stay within the safety limits of toxicity. Gentamicin blood levels must be checked, especially if the renal function is impaired.

Pseudomonas infections are especially difficult to overcome and are often sensitive only to a small group of antibiotics, e.g. cephalosporins, the majority of which can only be given by injection. Try to use the parenteral antibiotics in hospitals and to reserve the very few oral drugs, e.g. Uticillin for domiciliary use, if needed.

Intravesical instillation of chlorhexidine 1 in 5000 or Noxyflex 2.5% may be used for severe or recalcitrant bladder infections. For outpatient use, Urotainer with chlorhexidine instillation is a valuable adjunct to an indwelling catheter.

A high fluid intake should be encouraged, since the washout effect of a diuresis and the frequent bladder emptying that results is of major value in eliminating a bacteriuria. Sodium bicarbonate or potassium citrate may help severe bladder symptoms.

In cases of recurrent infections radiological investigation of the renal tract is mandatory to exclude anatomical or pathological abnormalities. If such structural abnormalities are found, it is often necessary to correct them surgically before the infection can be fully eliminated.

In addition to the antimicrobial agents already mentioned, other drugs often and effectively used as first-line treatment are Septrin (trimethoprim 80 mg and sulphamethoxazole 400 mg) tab 2 b.d., ampicillin (Penbritin) 500 mg t.d.s., amoxycillin (Amoxil) 250 mg t.d.s., nitrofurantoin 100 mg t.d.s. and nalidixic acid (Negram) 1 g t.d.s., and cyprofloxacin (Ciproxin) 500 mg b.d.

In pregnancy ampicillin, Amoxil and Furadantin are the drugs of choice. Sulphonamides should not be used in the third trimester. Septrin and tetracyclines should be avoided totally.

16

Acute Septicaemia

The urinary tract is the commonest source of septicaemia (or bacteraemia). This is partially due to the very close proximity of the blood vessels to the urethelium. In certain areas of the urinary tract there is very little separating the two and, hence, it is not surprising that organisms pass readily through this thin barrier. It is therefore important that patients who are known to have a urinary tract infection be treated for that infection before operation and be given the relevant antibiotic with the pre-medication.

The commonest infecting agent is a Gram-negative microorganism, and many of the symptoms are due to the release of endotoxins from this Gram-negative bacillus. The presenting symptoms of septicaemia vary with the severity of the infections, and are usually (but not always) those of pyrexia with rigors, often associated with hypotension and tachycardia or occasionally, in severe cases, coma or oliguria. The patient has usually undergone some form of urethral manipulation very recently, although this is not always the case.

1. *This is a critical condition and you must act quickly*. Remember that the clinical picture may be complicated by post-operative haemorrhage and you must ascertain that the hypotension is not due to either blood loss or myocardial failure (possibly following a coronary thrombosis). An ECG may be necessary to exclude a myocardial infarction.
2. An intravenous infusion must be started, a blood culture must be taken and "best-guess" antibiotics must be started immediately. The offending organism is usually a Gram-negative bacillus, e.g. *E. coli*, *Aerobacter aerogenes*, *Proteus*, etc., and therefore a combination of gentamicin 120 mg and ampicillin 500 mg should be given intravenously as soon as the blood culture has been taken. Second-generation cephalosporins may be preferred, e.g. cefuroxime 1.5 g, although these are expensive drugs and have little extra to offer in these cases. Metronidazole 500 mg (for anaerobic organisms) may be required.
3. Careful monitoring of blood pressure and of urine output is

essential. If hypotension persists, oliguria may occur and acute renal failure may develop. It is essential to maintain adequate fluid intake, and a diuretic (Lasix) may be required to boost urine output. Hydrocortisone may be helpful in refractory cases.

4. In severe cases it will be necessary to establish a central venous line to monitor fluid balance. You should consider transferring the patient to the Intensive Care Unit.

5. Antibiotic therapy should be altered if cultures of urine or blood show that such a change is desirable.

17

Pre-operative Antibiotics

As has already been discussed, Gram-negative bacteria following operation on the urinary tract are very common and the consequences of such an infection may be extreme. It has been repeatedly demonstrated that prophylactic antibiotics in routine "clean" cases are of little or no value, but there are three groups of patients who are at additional risk and in whom, therefore, the use of pre-operative antibiotics is justified:

1. Those who have heart valve disease, artificial valves, artificial joints or vascular grafts, etc.
2. Those who have had a long-term indwelling catheter or nephrostomy tubes.
3. Those who are known to have an existing infection.

It is, therefore, desirable to provide prophylactic antibiotic cover for these patients during any urological procedure, and the following regimen is suggested:

Ampicillin 500 mg i.m. and gentamicin 80 mg i.m. given approximately 30 min before surgery. Gentamicin 80 mg is also given i.m. 8 h after the operation and again 8 h after that.

Ampicillin should be omitted if there is any suggestion of a penicillin hypersensitivity. Erythromycin 500 mg i.v. may be used in its place, if necessary.

18

Drugs Affecting Bladder Function

This subject is not, strictly speaking, a topic to be included in a text on emergency management, but it is a subject that is specific to the young doctor in urology and, therefore, merits a brief mention.

There has recently been much experimental work on the pharmacology of the function of the lower urinary tract. The advent and development of urodynamics has allowed careful objective observation to be carried out in large series of patients and volunteers. These studies have greatly advanced the understanding of many of the disorders of micturition and have helped to indicate how bladder, sphincter and urethral behaviour can be modified by the administration of a variety of drugs.

The studies also demonstrate how *very variable is the measured objective response to the drugs, how very variable are the symptoms of any given bladder dysfunction and how variable are the side-effects of the administered drugs*. Many of the drugs that are found to have a pharmacological effect on the bladder act at more than one site and therefore may produce more than one effect. Many of these secondary effects are undesirable and unacceptable to the patient.

The assessment of the effect of drugs on bladder behaviour is further complicated by the very clear fact that *there is often a very strong psychological element to bladder symptoms, and it is repeatedly evident that in any series concerning patient evaluation there is a very high placebo response rate*.

DETRUSOR INSTABILITY

The stable bladder fills without inducing a significant rise in intravesical pressure, until it has reached its normal maximum capacity. The unstable detrusor is one that contracts sporadically and spontaneously during this filling process. The symptoms this produces are usually those of frequency, nocturia, urgency and urge incontinence. The mechanism of detrusor instability is not fully understood and research has produced many interesting data and much descriptive jargon.

Instability may often be the result of demonstrable abnormalities, e.g. infection, bladder stone, prostatic obstruction, bladder tumours, etc., and therefore such pathology must be sought and, if present, treated. In those in whom no such abnormality is detected, drug therapy may be of value, although, as already explained, it may not always be effective.

1. Oxybutanin (5 mg t.d.s.). Probably the most effective. It has anti-cholinergic and smooth muscle relaxant properties (i.e. musculotrophic). May produce dry mouth, dizziness, sleepiness and blurring of vision, etc.
2. Micturin (25 mg b.d.). Has anticholinergic and calcium antagonist action. Dose may be increased until either it is effective or the anticholinergic side-effects are unacceptable.
3. Pro-Banthine (30–60 mg t.d.s.). This anticholinergic drug will almost certainly produce side-effects if it is to be of value to the bladder.
4. Emepromium bromide (Cetiprin) (200 mg t.d.s.). Anticholinergic action. On rare occasions can produce oesophageal ulceration.
5. Imipramine (50 mg t.d.s.). Anticholinergic together with muscle relaxant and anaesthetic effect.

DRUGS WHICH IMPROVE BLADDER EMPTYING

Any attempt to use drugs to overcome retention or to reduce residual urine must be preceded by a careful examination to identify and exclude organic outflow obstructive lesions. Drugs exhibiting a cholinergic effect may theoretically be expected to improve detrusor contractability and alpha-adrenergic blockade may be of help in decreasing outflow resistance. The following drugs have a variable degree of effectiveness:

1. Carbachol (2 mg t.d.s. or 250 µg subcutaneously). A cholinergic agonist. Increases the strength of detrusor contractions. May cause cholinergic side-effects, e.g. sweating, intestinal colic, blurred vision, etc.
2. Ubretid (5 mg b.d.). An anticholinesterase. May also lead to cholinergic side-effects.
3. Phenoxybenzamine (20–30 mg daily). An adrenergic blocker

which produces a decrease in outflow resistance. May cause severe hypotension and tachycardia. To be used with caution and in low doses initially.

4. Prazosin (2 mg increasing to 20 mg daily). Has alpha blocker effects which may produce an increased urine flow rate and reduces frequency. Similar side-effects to those of phenoxybenzamine.

5. Indoramin (Doralese 20 mg b.d.). Action similar to Prazosin.

Part III

In the Accident and Emergency Department

(The Initial Management)

19

The Referred Patient

The patients that you will be asked to see in the Accident and Emergency Department will be categorised eventually in accordance with a variety of diagnoses, but almost without exception the reason they are seeking emergency medical attention is because they are in pain, often severe pain. The pain of a ureteric colic, of a bladder stretched to twice its comfortable capacity or of an ischaemic testis is extreme and is usually compounded by apprehension, by fear and by a knowledge that there is nothing that the patient can do about it and that he or she must therefore rely on others.

Fortunately you are in a position to alleviate the distress and it is therefore an obligation and a kindness to do so as soon as you can. It is, of course, not always possible to be instantly available, *but you should regard your availability to this particular patient in pain as being a very high priority and to consider that perhaps the task to which you are currently committed may be less important and can be interrupted.*

A prompt, even if abbreviated, visit is of enormous psychological value to the patient. The realisation that someone is interested in and is taking note of their problem and is doing something about it makes a massive contribution to their well-being.

Most emergency patients will have with them a letter from their GP giving a brief account of the immediate problem, the relevant past history, current drug therapy, etc. These letters should be read carefully and due attention paid to the diagnosis and opinions expressed. Remember that many of the referring GPs are very experienced clinicians and that their diagnoses are usually correct. Unfortunately, there are also GPs who are less diligent. It is therefore essential that you reach your own conclusions.

A second group of patients on whom you are asked to give an opinion are those who have no referring letter but who have been brought to the Accident and Emergency Department by friends or relations because they have been involved in an accident or have developed an acute and dramatic symptom. Usually these patients will have been seen initially by the casualty officer on duty who will then call you if he feels that the problem is urological in nature.

Irrespective of the mode of referral to the Accident and Emergency Department, it becomes your task to make or confirm a preliminary diagnosis, to reassure the patient, and to arrange his immediate management, his discharge to his home or his transfer to the ward.

20

Common Acute Symptoms and Their Early Management

Urological symptoms as met with in the outpatient clinics tend to be very non-specific and it is often difficult to make an accurate diagnosis on the bases of signs and symptoms alone. However, the interpretation of the emergency clinical presentation is usually facilitated by the fact that the signs and symptoms are rather more dramatic: e.g. a distended painful bladder associated with an inability to pass urine obviously suggests urinary retention; a swollen painful testicle of sudden onset in a young boy must indicate the likelihood of a torsion and therefore make surgical exploration of the scrotum mandatory.

However, it is important to remember that the fact that you are a member of a urological team does not mean that the patient you are asked to see is necessarily suffering from a lesion of the renal tract. Always be aware of other acute abdominal emergencies that may masquerade as ureteric colic, urinary retention, etc.

It is not the purpose of this handbook to describe the clinical presentation of all urological emergencies, since this information can be obtained from textbooks and from experience. It may, however, be useful to outline very briefly the urological implications of some of the more common presenting symptoms, bearing in mind that exceptions are common and variation is enormous.

ABDOMINAL PAIN

1. Loin and iliac fossa pain suggest the possibility of renal or ureteric pathology, and although you may achieve a fairly confident diagnosis by listening and examining, it is rarely possible to know the exact nature of the problem without recourse to X-rays, etc., and the necessary investigations must be arranged.
2. Suprapubic pain, especially when associated with disorder of micturition, suggests bladder problems. Acute retention is, of

course, associated with other symptoms and with fairly obvious clinical signs.

Bladder infection, stones, etc., should also be considered but do not usually require to be admitted as emergencies. Arrangements should be made for initial investigation and treatment of these cases as outpatients and an appointment should be made at the urology clinic in the near future.

A stone at the lower end of the ureter may present with severe symptoms of bladder irritation; usually, however, there is or has been some iliac fossa or loin pain.

3. Epigastric, periumbilical and hypochondriacal pain are not commonly indicative of urological conditions and the opinion of the general surgeons may be required.

Beware the drug addict who enjoys pethidine and knows what symptoms to describe. These patients are often known to the staff of the Accident and Emergency Department.

TRAUMA

Usually the history indicates fairly clearly the part of the renal tract that may have been traumatised. Trauma is discussed in detail in Chapter 23.

Trauma to the external genitalia may be slight and therefore be dealt with adequately in the Accident and Emergency Department, or may require a general anaesthetic, exploration and suture as an inpatient. If in doubt, discuss the case with your seniors.

TESTICULAR PAIN

This usually indicates torsion or infection, but occasionally a lower ureteric stone may cause pain to be referred to the testicle. Trauma should also be considered although if this is the cause, the history is usually fairly clear.

HAEMATURIA

Passing blood in urine engenders great anxiety in the patient and should always be investigated. It may derive from any pathology of any part of the renal tract and is often the only presenting feature of urological malignancies.

If there is sufficient blood loss to cause difficulty with micturition, pain, clinical anaemia, etc., then these patients will require to be managed as inpatients. Painless haematuria of this magnitude usually is the result of bleeding from a bladder tumour or from prostatic blood vessels. If there is also loin pain or colic, renal pathology is more likely.

Often, however, the haematuria is relatively slight and can be investigated at outpatient level, in which case you should reassure the patient and arrange for an IVU to be performed in the very near future.

In every case of haematuria, initial investigation demands an urgent though not instant IVU, the estimation of haemoglobin, a full blood count, bleeding and clotting time, serum electrolytes and an MSU. Cystoscopy, further X-rays, scan, cytology, etc., may be required at a later date after the initial IVU has been examined.

NAUSEA AND VOMITING

These are not commonly presenting symptoms in urology but may occasionally accompany ureteric colic or suggest uraemia.

21

To Admit or to Investigate as an Outpatient

Each week patients are admitted to the wards when they do not in fact require immediate hospital treatment. This is a pity, since most people would prefer to be at home and because it results in the inefficient use of limited acute beds. However, it is always best to err on the side of safety and compassion. It is preferable to admit a patient unnecessarily than to send a patient home with a dangerous condition. If in doubt, discuss the case with your seniors. If it is decided that the patient should go home, you must:

1. Arrange an outpatient clinic appointment so that he or she may be reassessed at a later date.
2. Arrange any relevant investigations that can be done at outpatient level   before this clinic appointment.
3. Telephone the patient's family doctor to inform him or her of your decision and action.

22

Retention

Urinary retention is probably the commonest emergency condition that you will be called upon to deal with in the Accident and Emergency Department. Although retention can develop at any age and in both male and female, the usual patient is an elderly man who is in pain, and catheterisation should be performed as soon as possible.

Regardless of the specific abnormality that results in retention of urine, in general terms the condition develops when the outflow tract resistance is such that the bladder musculature cannot overcome it. Hence, it may occur in the following circumstances:

1. When the bladder neck or urethra is obstructed, e.g. by an enlarged prostate or stricture.
2. When the detrusor contractions are inadequate, e.g. in spinal cord injury, in M.S. or in the early post-operative period.
3. When a combination of the above circumstances exists.

In fact, acute retention is rarely a state that occurs spontaneously with a normal bladder. In almost every case subclinical chronic retention has existed for a variable period and the "acute" state may be precipitated by factors such as constipation, infection, general illness, etc.

Remember that although the patient may be sent to you with a diagnosis of acute retention, there are other conditions that can mimic retention and you must therefore make your own assessment and diagnosis. Common misdiagnoses include intestinal obstruction, ascites, pelvic masses, aortic aneurysm, peritonitis from appendicitis or from perforated ulcer, etc.

The commonest cause of urinary retention in general hospital practice is prostatic obstruction, but you must always be aware of the possibility of a urethral lesion such as stricture, stone or tumour and of conditions involving the central nervous system.

Rectal examination is essential. It allows you to form a clinical impression as to whether the prostate is benign or malignant and to obtain a rough estimate of its size, and, in the case of a malignancy, its stage. More importantly, it allows the detection of tumours of the rectum and anal canal which might present with micturition difficulties and the exclusion of faecal loading and constipation as a cause of the retention.

A false impression of the size of the prostate may be obtained if the rectal examination is performed before the bladder is drained. The gland may then appear larger than it really is, since the full bladder tends to push the prostate downwards and backwards into the rectum. The finding of a small or apparently normal prostate does not exclude it as a cause of retention, since examination of the outer aspect of the prostate does not indicate its effect on the prostatic urethra.

A hard prostate usually indicates malignancy, but a prostate containing many stones, a small fibrous prostate and a prostate invaded by a bladder tumour may all have a similar consistency and masquerade as a primary prostatic malignancy.

Retention in the female is relatively uncommon, and careful pelvic examination is required to detect mass lesions in the uterus, ovaries or vagina. Neuropathies and faecal impaction must be excluded.

Whatever the cause, acute retention of urine demands that the bladder be drained either by urethral or by suprapubic catheterisation.

Always record the volume of urine obtained by catheterisation. Always take a catheter specimen of urine and send it for bacteriological examination.

If the urine is cloudy or if the catheterisation is to any degree traumatic, it is wise to commence the patient on an oral antimicrobial agent.

Routine inpatient tests should include haemoglobin and full blood count; urea and electrolytes as an indication of renal function; prostatic tumour markers to suggest, confirm or exclude malignancy; chest X-ray; plain X-ray of the renal tract to identify renal or bladder calcification and to exclude bony metastases or other skeletal abnormalities. Other tests may be required later in individual cases, e.g. ECG, IVU if there has been a history of haematuria; ultrasound; bone scan; etc.

ACUTE RETENTION

This is common and is usually very painful. Relieve it as soon as possible. Do not waste time in extensive history taking or examination. Ask and examine just enough to confirm the diagnosis and to obtain relevant previous urological history. Then perform catheterisation without delay using a 14 Fr or 16 Fr latex Foley catheter. Rectal examination is normally not required until after the catheter has been passed and the patient is more comfortable.

CHRONIC RETENTION

Chronic retention *per se* does not commonly present to the Accident and Emergency Department, since it is not usually a painful condition. However, the condition may present because of a concomitant infection or because some other condition has drawn the GP's attention to it. The bladder may be grossly distended, easily seen and palpated. The patient may insist that he is passing urine as usual, although he may admit to incontinence (overflow incontinence). It would not be unreasonable to investigate these patients as outpatients provided that there are no complicating factors.

If, however, it is decided to admit them to the ward, then they should be catheterised in the usual way with the added precaution of decompressing the bladder relatively slowly, over perhaps an hour, using a gate clip on the catheter. Rapid drainage of a chronically distended bladder may occasionally produce unwelcome haematuria. These patients are often uraemic, and bladder drainage will improve their renal function. Their prostates are often quite small.

ACUTE ON CHRONIC RETENTION

This occurs, for example, in a patient who has for some years had chronic bladder outflow obstruction and has finally reached the state when he is unable to pass urine at all. The bladder is greatly distended but the patient may not be in great pain. Catheterise, using relatively slow decompression.

CLOT RETENTION

This is not commonly met in the Accident and Emergency Department. It may, however, occur in a patient who has recently had prostatic or bladder surgery and who has developed a secondary haemorrhage a week or two after leaving hospital. Sometimes the patient is known to have a bladder tumour or is known to have had radiotherapy to the bladder. Alternatively, the patient may be quite unknown and undiagnosed.

Regardless of the underlying condition, the retention may be produced by a relatively small clot that has blocked the outflow tract, thus causing retention of otherwise fairly clear urine, or may be due to a massive intravesical haemorrhage causing the bladder to fill with clot which cannot escape. In either case it is wise to catheterise with a three-way plastic irrigating catheter. A latex catheter is inadvisable, because suction on the catheter with a bladder syringe normally results in occlusion of the lumen; the plastic catheter, on the other hand, is relatively rigid and collapse does not occur. Clots should be removed by syringing and bladder irrigation should be started (see p. 26). Transfusion may be necessary. Antibiotics should be prescribed routinely, since infection is a common cause of secondary haemorrhage.

23

Trauma

It is probable that you will be called to the Accident and Emergency Department to give an opinion in a case of trauma where injury to the kidney, bladder or urethra is suspected. You will be expected to declare whether such an injury is likely and to initiate the correct management. If you feel that there may have been an injury to the urinary tract then it is essential that the site and extent of such an injury be correctly determined. The proper management, and therefore the prognosis, will depend on this assessment. Your task is to make the initial assessment and to arrange the relevant investigations. *Do not try to manage these cases without talking to more experienced members of the urology team.*

URETHRAL AND BLADDER INJURY

You should suspect a urethral or bladder injury if there has been a history of pelvic or perineal trauma associated with any of the following features:

1. Blood at the external urethral meatus.
2. Open injury to penis or perineum.
3. Haematoma or extravasation into the perineum, scrotum or penis.
4. Fracture of the bony pelvis, especially of the pubic rami. (The urethra passes through and is firmly fixed to the perineal membrane. This "membrane" is attached to the inferior pubic rami on either side and to the symphysis pubis in front. Any fracture or displacement involving these bones is therefore particularly liable to result in displacement of the perineal membrane and, hence, damage to the urethra.)

71

Injury to the Anterior Urethra

The anterior urethra is at risk when there has been trauma to the perineum or penis. Examination may reveal bruising, extravasation or laceration of the perineum, scrotum or penis, and there may be blood at the external meatus.

If this is an isolated and relatively minor injury and the patient is otherwise fit, it is reasonable to delay any intervention until he has attempted to pass urine in the usual way. If micturition occurs without difficulty, then no further treatment is necessary, although follow-up should be arranged. *If the patient cannot pass urine, you may try to pass a small-calibre latex urethral catheter, but if there is difficulty, you should wait until the bladder becomes palpable and then perform suprapubic catheterisation* (see p. 19). A urethrogram may be considered necessary at a later date.

If there is an open injury, the appropriate toilet and suture will, of course, be required. If there is massive haematoma formation and extravasation, drainage may be necessary.

Injury to the Posterior Urethra

Posterior urethral injuries should be suspected when there has been an injury to the pelvis, especially when there is a fracture of the pubic rami or dislocation of the pubic symphysis, or disruption of the pelvic girdle. *In many cases it may be difficult to know whether the injury is to the urethra, to the bladder or to both.* Often these patients have other severe injuries with major haemorrhage and are clinically shocked. Such injuries take priority in treatment, but when the clinical state is stabilised, it is essential that you establish the extent of the urethral or bladder injury as accurately as possible. Most cases fall into the following two groups.

IN VERY MINOR PELVIC TRAUMA

It is acceptable in cases of minor pelvic trauma to allow the patient to attempt to pass urine normally when he is ready to do so. If this is achieved, it is unlikely that there is significant injury and instrumentation is not required or desirable.

If the patient cannot pass urine and retention with a palpable bladder develops, it is permissible for you to attempt to pass a fine 12–14 Fr latex Foley catheter, using careful sterile technique and plenty of anaesthetic lubricant. Usually there will be no difficulty in draining the bladder and as a rule the urine obtained will be clear. *If it proves difficult or too painful to pass the urethral catheter, immediately use a suprapubic catheter provided that the bladder is palpable and urine can be aspirated.*

IN SEVERE PELVIC TRAUMA

These cases may possibly be associated with multiple fractures, abrasions, head injuries, flail chest, ruptured viscera, etc. If there are features which suggest that lower urinary tract damage may also have occurred, it is essential at an early stage that you *determine whether the injury is to the bladder, to the urethra or to both.* It is important also to determine whether a urethral injury is a partial or a complete transection. Remember that you must assess the patient as a whole and that co-operation with other surgical specialities is vital. Blood transfusion may be required and antibiotics should be used.

Physical examination of these severely injured patients is often extremely difficult. There is frequently so much abdominal pain, guarding and peritonism that it may be quite impossible to determine with certainty the presence or absence of a distended bladder, impossible clinically to be certain of the type of injury that has occurred, and therefore *dangerous to employ a suprapubic catheter without further information.* Attempting to differentiate between complete and incomplete transection of the urethra by rectal examination alone is unsatisfactory. This is often inaccurate, usually impracticable owing to other injuries, and always extremely painful for the patient. It is therefore an unnecessary and ill-advised manoeuvre.

This essential information, and therefore a guide to management, is best obtained by means of an ascending urethrogram, which can be easily performed during the course of radiological assessment of bony and other injuries.

A suggested technique of urethrography is as follows: A fine Foley catheter (10 Fr) is introduced into the distal 1 in of the urethra and the balloon is inflated sufficiently to occlude the urethra. A water-soluble, iodine-containing, radio-opaque medium (e.g. Hypaque, Urograffin) is then injected, without force, into the urethra. Ideally this would be done under image intensifier screening, but this is often impracticable, and static films are usually sufficient. In most cases anteroposterior films are adequate, but occasionally a lateral film may be necessary.

INTERPRETATION AND MANAGEMENT

1. If the Hypaque reaches the intact bladder without extravasation through the urethral wall, then there is no significant injury. A urethral catheter may be passed to facilitate future general management—urine output measurement, etc.

2. If the dye shows an intact urethra but extravasation occurs from the bladder, *a urethral latex Foley catheter is passed* to drain the bladder and is left in situ. This is sufficient in most cases of **extraperitoneal bladder damage**, although occasionally, if there is gross extravasation from the bladder, a paravesical drain may be required later. If the injury has caused an **intraperitoneal rupture of the bladder**, this will be demonstrated on the contrast X-ray. An attempt to use a suprapubic catheter would be dangerous, as the bladder will normally not be distended, since the urine readily leaks into the peritoneal cavity. Again *it is possible that a urethral catheter is all that is required*, but under these circumstances it is often necessary to perform a laparotomy to exclude injury to other organs, and at operation the tear in the bladder can be identified and sutured and the peritoneal cavity drained.

3. If the dye extravasates through the urethral wall but nevertheless also reaches the bladder, this suggests **a partial transection of the urethra** and *suprapubic catheterisation is required*. Wait until the bladder becomes palpable so that the procedure may be performed safely and efficiently. If there is gross perineal or scrotal extravasation and haematoma formation, a perineal drain may be required later.

4. If the dye extravasates from the urethra and does not reach the bladder, then **a complete transection of the urethra** has probably occurred, usually at the membranous urethra. *Open operation is required*, to remove the resulting haematoma and to align the torn ends of the urethra. This is done in theatre by an experienced member of the urology team. *Suprapubic catheterisation is required as a temporary means of draining the distended bladder*, until resuscitation of the patient has been completed and he is fit for open surgery.

RENAL INJURY

Injury to the kidney should be suspected if there has been trauma to the back, upper abdomen or loin, followed by haematuria. If the renal injury is minor, haematuria may be the only presenting feature. If there has been major trauma, there may also be extravasation of blood or urine into perirenal tissues presenting as a loin swelling.

Management will, of course, also depend on the general state of the patient, but, assuming this to be satisfactory, you should request an IVU. The purpose of this X-ray is, first, to confirm the presence and condition of a kidney on the unaffected side and, second, to indicate in general terms the nature and severity of the injury to the affected kidney. Interpretation of the IVU in trauma is difficult, but usually there is time for you to discuss this with the radiologist and your surgical colleagues. Urgent surgical treatment is rarely indicated.

Initial treatment is usually by conservative means. Analgesics are important, since there may be associated bony injury to rib, transverse processes, spine, etc. Clot colic may be another source of pain. The patient should be admitted for careful observation. Blood transfusion may be required. Antibiotics should be prescribed.

Active intervention would be considered at an early stage only if there was increasing loin swelling together with a clinical state suggesting unremitting haemorrhage.

At a later stage retrograde X-rays, isotope scans and angiography may be indicated to help to decide whether operative intervention would be useful, but the decision to order such investigations will be taken by your seniors. *Initially your aim should be to resuscitate, to control pain and to ensure adequate overall renal function.*

24

Epididymo-orchitis and Torsion of Testis

You will often find it very difficult to differentiate between these two conditions. *If there is any reasonable doubt, exploration of the scrotum should be performed.* No harm will be done by exploring an infected scrotum but a great deal of harm may be done by *not* exploring a torsion.

The following points may be helpful in reaching a diagnosis but they are not to be regarded as rules or apodictic. Each condition may mimic the other.

In cases of *infection* the patient tends to be relatively older, the onset of symptoms is usually fairly gradual and there may be a history of urethral instrumentation. The epididymis may be palpable and tender, the patient may be constitutionally unwell and there is often a urinary tract infection. Pyrexia is usual.

Patients with *torsion* of the testicle are usually in a much younger age group. Many of the patients are children or young adults. Often the history is of a sudden onset of pain, possibly, but not invariably, associated with physical exercise. The testis may lie horizontally and high in the scrotum. It is the testis that is tender rather than the epididymis. The patient is not pyrexial and has a sterile urine.

You must remember that other conditions such as strangulated inguinal hernia, scrotal haematoma following injury, torsion of an appendix, testis or idiopathic scrotal oedema, should also be considered.

There is no time limit on the need to operate on a suspected torsion. The scrotum should be explored as soon as the patient is fit for anaesthesia, since the degree of ischaemia produced by obstruction of the blood supply varies from case to case. At one end of the spectrum, ischaemia is immediate and complete and the testicle will infarct very rapidly. At the other end, the ischaemia may be partial only, and the situation therefore may be reversible long after first symptoms become apparent.

When operating on a suspected torsion, try always to preserve the testicle rather than remove it. Although spermatogenesis may have been jeopardised, the hormonal function is normally intact. Remember to "fix" *both* testicles by suturing the tunica to the overlying scrotal layers.

Remember also to explain to the patient that although an attempt will be made to preserve the testicle, it may be necessary to perform an orchidectomy.

In a case of orchitis always be aware that there may be a testicular tumour lurking under the infection, and it is sensible therefore to estimate testicular tumour markers in each case. It is often unnecessary to admit these patients to the ward. Their essential requirements are antibiotics, scrotal support, analgesics and rest, all of which can be obtained at home. Uncommonly, scrotal drainage is required if the infection does not respond to antibiotics and pus forms, in which case the GP, who should be informed of the intention to send the patient home, will return him to the hospital. Always ensure that the patient returns to outpatients after the infection subsides, so that the testicle can be properly examined. Ultrasound of the testicle may be valuable.

25

Renal or Ureteric Colic

The pain experienced as a calculus passes from the renal pelvis to the bladder may be extremely severe or it may be a mere discomfort. The degree of pain is unrelated to the size of the stone but is due mainly to ureteric spasm and, to a lesser extent, to the ureteric and calyceal distension secondary to the obstruction.

Although the commonest cause of ureteric colic is the presence of a stone, colic may also be produced by other obstructive lesions within or outside the ureter: for example, congenital pelviureteric obstruction, clot colic, ureteric tumour, and occasionally, retroperitoneal fibrosis or extraureteric tumours, etc.

These latter conditions will not be demonstrated on a plain X-ray and it is therefore always useful in a case of renal or ureteric pain to obtain an IVU as soon as possible. This X-ray will suggest the cause and indicate the site and the severity of the obstruction. Usually only one or two radiographs are necessary. It will also enable you to ascertain that the patient's pain is indeed due to a ureteric colic and not due to other dangerous intra-abdominal conditions, such as appendicitis, biliary colic, perforated ulcer, twisted ovarian cysts, ectopic pregnancy, leaking aneurysm, etc. An IVU is important also to confirm the presence and state of the contralateral kidney.

Analgesics should be given in adequate doses. Most adults will require 100 mg pethidine, and if the patient is on the large size or appears to be in severe pain, you should not hesitate to prescribe 150 mg pethidine. Antispasmodics may help and rarely do harm. Be aware also that there are some patients who know that if they simulate renal colic, they will probably be given pethidine or other narcotic. These patients are relatively few and are often known to the Accident and Emergency Department.

Ensure that there is no urinary infection or pyrexia. Prescribe antibiotics if there is.

It is rare for ureteric or renal obstruction to require instant surgical relief but there are occasions when this would be essential and it is important that these occasions be recognised.

1. When the affected ureter is severely obstructed and the contra-lateral kidney is either absent or functioning very poorly.
2. When both ureters are obstructed, although the presenting symptoms may be derived from only one side.
3. When there is, in addition to the pain of ureteric colic, a pyrexia with rigors indicating the probable presence of infection above the obstructing stone (pyonephrosis).

In these circumstances it is important to bypass or remove the obstruction without delay. This may be achieved by various means, e.g. percutaneous nephrostomy, cystoscopy and ureteric catheterisation or, in the case of a stone, endoscopic removal. *It is vital that these cases be identified and discussed with your seniors, who will decide when and how the case is to be dealt with.*

Many ureteric calculi (90%) will pass spontaneously, given time, and therefore most patients can be treated conservatively. Many of these patients do not need to be admitted to the ward once a dignosis has been established and the obstructing stone has been assessed as one that will very likely be passed without surgical intervention. These patients can be sent home and an outpatient appointment appointment can be arranged. If, however, it is decided to admit the patient for diagnosis and observation, serum electrolytes, urea and creatinine, and a full blood count, should all be estimated, and an MSU should be examined. Analgesics should be prescribed and all urine should be sieved before being discarded. The stone risk factors are estimated and, if necessary, progress X-rays are arranged. It is not necessary to confine these patients to hospital until the stone is passed, and they may be allowed home when their symptoms subside.

26

Intravenous Urography

Intravenous or excretary urography is the mainstay in the investigation of most surgical conditions of the upper renal tract. It is an essential part of the investigation of haematuria and is usually required when investigating loin pain, chronic urinary infections, trauma, etc.

Most radiodiagnostic departments are, with good reason, fairly strict about the indications for an IVU, and a good case must be made when requesting such a time-consuming, expensive and potentially dangerous X-ray. It is important to indicate clearly to the radiologist what it is that you hope to gain by the X-ray and what the possible diagnosis might be. In this way the need for oblique views, for tomography, for delayed films, etc., may be anticipated and a much more relevant and reliable report be given. It is also a point of courtesy to your colleagues, who have a valuable expertise which is essential to you as part of the investigation and management of your patient.

The dangers of an IVU are derived from three sources: first, the repeated exposure to ionising radiation, e.g. in young patients or in patients who may have had many X-rays previously; second, the risk to the potentially pregnant patient, with whom the "ten day rule" must be strictly observed; and third, the possibility of a hypersensitivity or an anaphylactic reaction to the intravenous dye.

If, as occasionally occurs, it becomes your task to inject the contrast medium for a urogram, the following precautions should be observed.

1. Only low-osmolarity contrast media (e.g. Omnipaque, Niopam) should be used—this greatly reduces the likelihood of an anaphylactic reaction.
2. You should remain with and observe the patient for at least 20 min after the injection of the contrast, so that if a reaction does occur, it can be treated immediately. A feeling of flushing, nausea and sickness is a common occurrence after injections of radio-opaque dye and does not indicate a sensitivity reaction.

3. You should check the location in the X-ray Department of any emergency drug that may be necessary to combat a severe reaction, i.e. adrenaline, steroids, etc.

INTERPRETATION

It is important that you become proficient at reading the urogram series. The X-rays should be scrutinised in the order in which they were taken, starting with the control film.

When studying the *control film*, you should direct your attention first to the bones. Is there any congenital abnormality visible? Are there any fractures, narrowed disc spaces, osteophytes? Is the structure of the bones uniform and normal, and are there signs of metastases, of osteoporosis, of Paget's disease, of spondylitis, etc? Does the patient suffer from arthritis of hip joints? Second, your attention should be given to soft tissue shadows, e.g. psoas shadow, possible fluid collections, bladder outline, renal outline, bowel gas, etc. Finally, examine the renal, ureteric, bladder and prostatic areas for calcification. Are there gallstones visible? Is there pancreatic calcification? calcified fibroids? phleboliths?

Studying the *excretory phase* of the X-ray series in the proper order provides information about the function, the structure and the drainage of the kidneys. Aptitude in interpreting these features comes with experience, instruction and discussion. You should learn as soon as possible to recognise the normal renal outline and nephrogram, and learn the appearances of normal calyces and their papilla. Be able to identify a normal ureter, its size and its course. Learn to understand the significance of the cystogram phase of the IVU which should be seen both in the pre- and post-micturition films.

Only when you have a reasonable acquaintance with the appearances of a normal IVU will you be able to give a worth-while opinion of the abnormal. The more X-rays you see and discuss, the greater will be your ability to interpret abnormal appearances.

Index